BOOK ENDORSEMENTS

"R.J. Harris is a food addict who lost 200 pounds. He has written an inspiring book about that weight loss, that combines common sense with honesty and humor. It's a quick read that will have long-lasting effects for anyone who wants to lose weight and gain control of their life. I recommend it highly."

—Carmen Finestra, Co-creator of TV's *Home Improvement*

"The best part was how you lost the weight—exercise, moderation and eating healthy—the keys to it all. Thanks for being an inspiration to so many people. You have a gift that's worth sharing."

—Lori Burkholder, News Anchor for WGAL TV8, Lancaster, PA

"Weight is something every female and/or male thinks about if not fears. Whether it's 5lbs or 50lbs it's in our mind. Your book embraces the realistic side of what we all think, yet forget to practice. The touch of current events and childhood memories was extremely relatable but the point of changing your lifestyle is something that can't be ignored! JOB WELL DONE!"

—Holly Love, Air Personality, BOB 94.9 Radio, Harrisburg, PA

RADIO LISTENER QUOTES

"I stopped weighing myself at 365, and now my scale reads 205. I can't wait until I go under 200! When I listened to your story in the morning, I didn't believe it would be possible for me, but I am there!"

—Dan

"I lost 76 lbs since just doing the things you talk about every day. Thanks."

—Ernie

"You really are an inspiration and I truly commend your efforts and appreciate your journey."

—Marti

"Watching your video was very inspirational. It brought me to the realization that it is possible for me to get out of this rut and back on track again."

—Joanne

"Your personal struggle with weight loss has been an inspiration for those like me to keep plugging along with the ultimate target of reaching our own goal."

—David

It Ain't Easy

BEING FAT
But That's Your *Problem*

Tough Love from a
Recovering Overeater

It Ain't Easy

BEING FAT

But That's Your *Problem*

Tough Love from a
Recovering Overeater

R.J. Harris

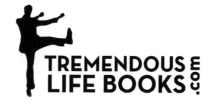

It Ain't Easy Being Fat, But That's Your Problem
Published by
Tremendous Life Books
206 West Allen Street
Mechanicsburg, PA 17055

ISBN: 978-1-933715-90-2

Book Production Services Provided by Gregory A. Dixon
Printed in the United States of America

The information provided in this book should not be construed as personal medical advice or instruction. Always consult a physician before beginning any diet program or fitness regimen. No action should be taken based solely on the contents of this book.

Readers should consult appropriate health professionals on any matter relating to their health and well being.

The information and opinions provided here are believed to be accurate and sound, based on the best judgment available to the author, but readers who fail to consult appropriate health authorities assume the risk of any injuries. The author and publisher are not responsible for errors or omissions.

All trademarks are property of their respective owners.

DEDICATION

I dedicate this book to the millions who suffer daily from addictive compulsive overeating.

TABLE OF CONTENTS

ACKNOWLEDGEMENTS

I t *Ain't Easy Being Fat, But That's Your Problem: Tough Love from a Recovering Overeater* has been a true joy to write. The thought of helping just one reader beat the addiction to food has made it a real pleasure. Without the love and support of family, friends, and listeners, my journey would have been impossible.

I would like to thank my wife Bonnie in particular. Her steadfast support over the decades has been my key to success. A recent medical study indicated that the one thing that your child learns from you and takes with them through their entire life is his eating habits. I thank God my children have their mother's eating habits. Thanks to my children Mike, Eric, Christi, and daughter-in-law

Lauren for being my biggest cheerleaders and believing that this time it was the real deal, and special love to my granddaughters Lydia and Leah, for they were the true inspiration for my weight loss. At their young age they only know a 400 pound me from photos of when Grandpop was fat.

Thanks to Tracy Turek-Wiley for her diligence in editing this book for me. I would also like to thank my good friends and brothers in Christ, Joe Fiedler and Charles "Tremendous" Jones for their incredible encouragement. Charles went home to the Lord on October 16, 2008. I miss him greatly. Thank you to the hundreds of WHP 580 listeners who have taken the time to write, call, and encourage me at live events. Your encouragement was the fuel for my rocket.

R.J. Harris

FOREWORD

Thomas Edison said, "Restlessness and discontent are the first necessities of progress." R.J.'s book is a clear reflection of this, showing how one man's refusal to continue down his current path of obesity led him to fully appreciate his greatest asset—his body.

R.J. chronicles his tremendous weight loss journey, providing tools for each of us to introduce and to use in our own lives. This book's true transforming power is based on the fact that it was written with simplicity and tough love.

There is only one way to lose weight....eat below your daily caloric needs. No fad diets, magical drinks and powders, or disciplined exercise regimes will change this basic truth.

R.J. is well aware of the hold food demons can have on us. Just like any other additive force, the demon of food can do just as much damage as the demon of drink, sex, or drugs.

But after reading his story of how he fought the battle and won, and seeing his continuing successes, you too will never consider a quick fix, trendy diet, or cosmetic surgery to deal with an issue that you can solve yourself.

Charlie "Tremendous" Jones

CHILDHOOD: THE DOOR TO OBESITY

In order to bring you to where I am today, we have to start around 1964 at age ten in the 300 block of Locust Street in Reading, Pennsylvania. I grew up in a diverse neighborhood that was once all Pennsylvania German, commonly referred to as Pennsylvania Dutch. As a result, my childhood diet was meat and potatoes, period. The only vegetables that we ate were corn and potatoes. I remember a kid at school talking about his mother washing lettuce for salad in the kitchen sink. I thought, "Wash lettuce? I didn't know that you had to do that." We never ate the stuff. Every piece of meat that we ever consumed was fried in crisco in an old cast iron frying pan. Crisco was a staple.

For the longest time I'd tell folks that I was as skinny as a rail until my teens, about the time that I became interested in radio. Truth is that is was more like ten. I proudly brag of my second grade photo that has me smiling and small enough that a good winter wind could blow me away. By fourth grade my caloric intake had already caught up with me, and by sixth grade I was well on my way to becoming a fat human being. My two best friends in life were also obese, "The Three Amigos" of eating.

Like many other fat kids, I was the last picked to play sports or for most any competition in gym class. The only thing that I was great at was archery, because I was a young hunter. My sports experience was relegated to playing baseball or football in the street or at a local park. Even then, I was never a key player. I still cherish the memory of being given the football while playing a game in the snow and scoring a touchdown. They gave me the ball because nobody ever suspected that I'd score.

At age twelve, I woke up one day and decided that I wanted to be a radio disc jockey. Electronics and radio gizmos became my hobby, leading to ham radio, and a career in commercial radio at age fourteen. I thought, like many others, that sitting on my butt was what helped me become fat. Instead of playing and running around, I sat all day talking to people via radio; however, all of the running around that I could do in a day would still not off-set the number of calories that I consumed. By that time three to four colas per day were the norm, along with potato chips, penny candy, and a few snack cakes for good measure. Add those calories to three or four pork chops fried in crisco with tasty fat on the edges, some corn and potatoes, and I had consumed a few thousand calories easily.

THE FIRST DIET

In eleventh grade I went on my first diet. I did not have or follow a plan. I just consumed less food. By that I mean I ate one pork chop fried in crisco rather than three or four, and I added applesauce to the mix. Yes, that was the one fruit that we'd eat occasionally. Did you catch that? I dieted… and lost weight by consuming RED MEAT fried in crisco! This tidbit is an important one and will come into play later on. I lost a lot of weight. So much so that my fat buddies were jealous, and one of them was determined to give me a run for my money. Shortly thereafter, I fell off the wagon and regained my weight—and then some. He did exactly the same. The first of many diet roller coaster rides to come.

My brother Rob joined a car club about the

time that I was looking my best. I joined the club and met the lady who would become my wife. Bonnie was so cute and thin. I was attracted to her, but really didn't think that I had much to offer. She was two years older and many of the good looking guys in the club had a far better chance than I. In short order I was elected vice-president of the club, and Bonnie was elected assistant secretary. That put us in a position to work closely with each other. After she had a chance to know me, my goals, my vision for life, and my sense of humor, we dated. We married on my eighteenth birthday, November 11, 1972.

Bonnie has always been thin. I proudly boast today that she can still wear her wedding dress. She always weighs 118-122 pounds. Even having our three children, she never put on much weight. Food has never driven her like it did me. Bonnie naturally eats healthy foods, along with the sweets that she likes, all in moderation. I thank God for Bonnie and her influence on our children. Our three kids have excellent eating habits and maintain a healthy weight because of their mother's influence, not mine.

My second diet came in our first year of marriage after we moved to Lebanon, Pennsylvania where I took a radio job. I joined Weight Watchers. This was my first experience with a commercial diet, although I was familiar with the program as my mother attended Weight Watchers on and off over a few decades. This was the first time that I was exposed to a healthy eating program. Oddly enough, if I would have been eating like my young bride, I'd have lost weight and been thin all along. I had several spells over the next couple of years of trying to lose weight on my own. Never achieving a lasting result, I always put the pounds that I lost back on and a few more for good measure.

In 1974 I took my first radio management job in Carlisle, Pennsylvania. Again I was gaining weight, when the owner of the restaurant next door suggested that I see this "diet doctor" just north of Harrisburg. No appointment was necessary. I drove up the next day, only to find people lined up out the door. I figured that I would never get in, turned around and went home. When I related this story the next day, the restaurant owner told me that it would have taken just minutes. I headed back up; while it was not as busy as the night before, the waiting room was still full. Within ten minutes I was seeing the doctor. He asked me why I was there. After stating that I wanted to lose weight, he handed me three bags of pills. That was it. I was rather naïve when it came to drugs, particularly pills. At age four I took a pouch full of my father's blood pressure medicine and had to have my stomach pumped. Until age eighteen no one could get me to take a pill, so I had no clue as to what speed was. I lasted one day on the doctor-prescribed diet pills. I could not sleep and at one point left our apartment to go vacuum the entire radio station. Never again would I take diet drugs. That doctor was arrested over a decade later and lost his license.

At the young age of twenty, my career took me to Philadelphia. I was cocky enough to say that I would make it to a major market by age 21. This is a big achievement for a radio personality, as Philly was the fourth largest market in the country at the time. It was those kinds of goals that Bonnie was attracted to. My car was really advanced for its time. Like the Lexus on the market today, my car could drive itself. Every night at 11:30 PM, it would automatically pull into Dunkin' Donuts in Phoenixville, Pennsylvania. Yes, automatically. Further, it would not start again unless I went in and made a purchase. This was back in the old days when I had to get out of my car and WALK both ways to get donuts. We didn't have the ease of a drive-thru. Honestly, my weight never got in my way. In radio, it was all about how good you are on the air. But I was still fat… and growing fatter. An ad for Overeaters Anonymous piqued my interest. I attended a meeting and was moved. People who understood, people who could identify, a sponsor to call when I want to eat three donuts with my coffee on the way to work.

Overeaters Anonymous helped me a great deal, for a while. They opened my eyes to the fact that I was addicted to food, like an alcoholic is to booze. The difference is that we cannot give up food like addicts can alcohol, drugs, or cigarettes. People completely abstain from those substances; food is a requirement!

The OA train ride ended when I took a radio management job in Harrisburg, Pennsylvania. I searched for an OA meeting before ever arriving in town. When I discovered that OA did not have a chapter in the area, a friend and I started one. The meetings were tough because I was the only one who had experienced the discipline of the program. The new folks turned the meetings into a tea party obsessing over the foods that they loved but could not have. Losing interest I exited and put pounds back on.

In 1977 came the first radio diet. Over the years I have done them all. No, I mean it. Hard to name one of the commercial diets that radio folks plug that I haven't been on.

I've endorsed Nutrisystem five times, also the Diet Workshop, Jenny Craig, LA Weight Loss, Body Solutions and more. Nutrisystem was the first, and I did the original, all liquid protein diet. I did not eat as much as a crumb for 34 days. I lost a lot of weight and felt fine. But I put all of those pounds back… and more.

Does any of this sound familiar to you? I bring you through this blow-by-blow chronology to illustrate what most of us experience. I always say that all diets work; it is a matter of sticking to them. The benefit that I had with all of these programs is learning about nutrition. After attending as many classes as I had over the years, I could teach nutrition. This information would come in handy once I really decided to make a change for life.

My next serious attempt to lose weight was in 1983 in Milwaukee. I did a radio endorsement deal while I was renovating almost every inch of our home. The distraction of remodeling kept me busy, and I made it down to 218! An amazing weight for me, given that I now hovered at about 300. I even became a certified soccer referee for my son Michael's under eight league. You already know what happened next. I gained all of those pounds back again … and a few more. Each time this happens, I set a new high-water mark.

The next two and a half decades I spent countless months on various diets that I endorsed on the radio, losing weight each time, gaining it right back, along with an extra ten or twenty pounds, diets of my own doing in between that lasted as lit-tle as a few hours. Once I screwed up a day, I was finished. I ate more and more, committing to resuming my diet tomorrow. Only tomorrow never came. It's amazing the silly roadblocks that we put in our own way. A universal one is that we never start a diet mid-week or on a weekend. Diets can only begin on a Monday. Monday, like tomorrow, never comes.

When we diet, it's like we place a weight over our heads, just waiting for it to come crashing down. Human beings have short attention spans and unrealistic goals. Even the heaviest eaters among us put on about twenty pounds per year. Yet if we do not take off that same twenty pounds in three weeks, we fail. We start diets that have us doing things that cause us to crash in short order. At the top of the list is getting by on foods that we do not particularly care for, followed by drinking an absurd amount of water daily. Let me get this straight: in order to lose weight I have to eat plenty of bland stuff and I have to feel like I have to pee 24/7? How long do you really think it will be before the weight over my head smacks me dead-on?

HITTING BOTTOM

L ike an alcoholic, I firmly believe that compulsive overeaters have to bottom out before they can straighten out. And just like an alcoholic, sometimes compulsive overeaters insist that they have bottomed out, when in fact, there is more out-of-control eating to come. Like most, I remember exactly where I was on September 11, 2001. The news of the World Trade Center terrorism hit us in a big way at the radio station. All ears were on WHP, as we were not only number-one rated, but the big news and information station as well. But vivid in my mind was my trek between Holy Spirit Hospital and the station as I was having tests done to get to the bottom of a nausea that would not go away. I was on the Atkins diet at the time and peeling off three to five pounds per week.

I had lost eighty pounds and the weight just kept coming off. God bless Doctor Atkins! Did I mention that I was nauseous?

I started my medical tests mid-day on 9/11; it seemed as if they would add another test soon after finding nothing with the one just completed. By afternoon the hospital was filled with fine Americans who just showed up to give blood, so many that folks had to be turned away. I will never forget the sight! It was two days later when I reported for a stress test that the cardiologist on duty noticed that my heart was racing and in irregular rhythm, and we had not even started the test. I was admitted immediately with atrilfibulation. Just one day later it was discovered that the same disorder that rocked my mother as a young girl, and caused her amazing rapid weight gain, would now be mine to deal with as well: hypothyroid disease. My thyroid would have to be killed off by radiation, and I would take replacement hormones the rest of my life. I was also told that I would not be in a position to lose weight for a time, as my metabolism would be super-slow until they found the right dose. This was my excuse to go on the final binge! I gained every one of those eighty pounds back and added nearly twenty more. Here we go again!

I ate everything that was not nailed down and hid any evidence of the binge eating. There was ten bucks worth of candy and junk food wrappers in a bag under my car seat at any given time. I had to eat outside the home. No way did I want my family to see this, even though they knew it was going on. My wife had discovered the wrappers, bags, or loose itemized receipts more than once, and the pounds had to be the result of more food than I had access to at home. The itemized receipt was the worst thing to happen to binge eaters. Now I had to be creative when slipping a couple of candy bars on the bill while getting groceries at the wife's direction. Bonnie scrutinized each receipt.

You should know that I loved every minute of binging! I joke that the owner of the vending machine at work had to declare bankruptcy over the loss of my revenue after I straightened out. At least three items for breakfast each morning came from that machine. I was so obsessed that I became angry when he continually placed lame items in it instead of the more popular peanut butter cups. My first love is peanut butter Easter eggs, a taste I acquired as a kid. I ate six at a time!

I love it when I run into a person who declares that no matter what he eats, he cannot gain weight. Let me put him on the "R.J. System." If he does not gain wait, I'll give him his money back. But he has to follow my program exactly, and he has to be able to eat six peanut butter eggs at a time, minimum! Use my system and he will gain weight.

People often ask what my ideal weight is. My ideal weight would be 1,007 pounds. That would give me the ability to eat whatever I want to. I have to pack away a lot of peanut butter Easter eggs and Tastykakes to achieve and maintain that level of girth.

Time went by and I was now at close to 400 pounds. Size fifty-eight pants were very tight, a sixty-inch waist was coming fast. Sixty-inches! Simple things were now difficult or impossible. All shoes were slip-on, even sneakers with laces. Tying shoes was not an easy task. To pick up the newspaper in the driveway I had to balance on one leg. I looked like one of those gravity operated birds that dipped for water. If I did not have a shovel or fence to help pull me up while gardening, I was not getting up. I actually purchased and started to use a pair of those long handled grabbers. What's next, a scooter chair? Look around, many of the folks in these power chairs are much too young to be in them, and most are grossly obese. I spent much of my waking time knowing that I had to stop, while continuing to gorge.

Other than being fat, my life was actually pretty darn good. The description was fitting for the opening of Wheel of Fortune: I had a wonderful and beautiful wife, three great children, a lovely daughter-in-law, and two beautiful grand daughters. WHP and my morning show were at the top of the heap in the Arbitron ratings, with one of the highest shares of any talk station nationwide. But I was still nearly 400 pounds! Was it time for drastic action?

A few years earlier I had talked with my doctor about stomach surgery. He said that the procedure was still relatively new and that I should wait two years or so, to see if I really wanted to do it. That would give the procedure some time to establish a record. Three years had now gone by, I had lost a lot of weight with Atkins, only to pack it and more back on; perhaps it was time.

Two things struck me: the mortality rate was still high and I noticed that some folks who had lost a lot of weight were now gaining it back. I thought, for some this is just another diet, but a radical one. I would be stuck with these physical changes for life. I told a few doctor friends that I felt that gastric bypass patients regaining their weight would be a big media story in the future. They responded by saying that they were already seeing it. In fact, at the time that this was written, my personal physician told me that he had ten patients who had had surgery. Eight had gastric bypass, while two had the laparoscopic gastric band procedure. Eight out of eight gastric bypass patients had lost weight (but not all that they had to lose) and had begun to gain weight again. They learned to eat around the bypass, a program that only treated the symptoms of this addiction. The two who had the band surgery were doing well.

While surgery works for some, I did not want to be one that went all that way, only to fail. One of the doctors told me that in order for the surgery to succeed, I would have to change the way I eat for life. I thought, if that was the case, why have the surgery? Just change!

At this point I was close to the bottom. I had no way of knowing exactly how much I weighed unless I went to a doctor—We didn't have a scale that would read that high. I do know that size fifty-eight pants were now too small and that I should have been wearing sixties. Can you image, a sixty-inch waistline?

While the employees were very nice, I hated every minute of having to shop at a big and tall store. It started when I was a kid. Nothing ever came off the shelf; I had to wear adult pants with the leg lengths hemmed by a friend's mom. Now I would have to go to the "fat guy store" for size sixty pants. Can 4X shirts be far behind? Something had to give. I was sick of being fat, tired of eating, but knew that any diet would be a challenge. It's hard to hold straight for fifty or seventy-five pounds; I now had over 200 to lose! I knew that I had a decision to make: either remain fat and try to manage the amount that I am overweight, or change forever. I thought long and hard about the first option. After all, forever is a long time.

One evening I was watching a local TV newscast. There was a heartbreaking flood story of a grandparent who was in a raging creek barely grasping his grandchild. The current was too strong and swept the child away to his death. It made me think of my granddaughters. I came to the conclusion that I could not save them, because I could not save myself. How could I save anyone when I am not fit enough to get off of my knees without a prop? That was the turning point, the bottom for me. I had subjected myself and my loved ones to this for far too long, and it was going to end!

THE PLAN

The U.S. Government says that people have used more than 28,000 ways to lose weight. Only one works. Eat the amount of food that God intended us to eat! Well I knew what I did not want to do: diet. If I have to change forever, do it. From now on I would eat a well-balanced food plan, based purely on what I enjoy. That also meant embracing fruits and vegetables that I truly enjoyed, but eagerly casting aside fattening alternatives. Utilizing all of the good nutrition from all of those diets that I was on, I would forge a calorie plan that would allow me to take off weight consistently. I did not care whether that meant one pound or three pounds per week. As long as I was going down and not going crazy, I'd be happy. But I knew that I needed help. Praying to the Lord was at the top of the order. You have no idea how often I turned to God, and still do, when the food demons came calling for me. I also found a need for support. I thought of Overeaters Anonymous and Weight Watchers immediately. While Overeaters Anonymous is a fine organization and helps many, I just could not see myself changing forever while obsessing over every morsel of food that goes into my mouth, or calling a sponsor when the food demons come for me. It worked for many, but for me it would be far from leading a "normal" existence with eating. I have always known that Weight Watchers was the most sensible of the weight loss programs that I have ever been on. They just so happened to have a meeting at 10:30 AM on Sunday morning. I would take in early church, then go weigh in. It was perfect! In the past, weekends were my toughest time. I knew that if I made it to Sunday morning that I would make it through the weekend!

Weight Watchers helped in two ways: account-ability and their Points plan. Their Points plan made what I was already determined to do easy. I was diligent about the count being right, and I wrote everything down, every day. Seeing Deanna and Barb at the weigh-in was the highlight of my week. I referred to them as my "probation officers." I looked at them as exactly that. For now I had to report each week, but eventually I would be a free man, on my own to make the right decisions. What did not work for me was their meetings. I stayed for just two. The leader/lecturer did an excellent job; it was the people in the class that caused me not to attend. They sat around obsessing over what they could not have and little nonsensi-cal shortcuts to get around calories. I wanted to stand up and say, "You people don't get it and will be here off and on for life if you don't wise up!" But I had just started and had not accomplished anything yet.

The point system easily allowed me to eat at Applebee's, Burger King, Dunkin' Donuts, local diners, and my favorite Philly cheese steak place. But I also embraced fresh fruits and vegetables, along with more poultry, fish, and turkey. I ate an ice cream dessert along with a healthy serving of pretzels every evening. Oh, except Saturday when I had a strawberry sundae from Dairy Queen. Eating what I enjoyed was the only way that I could change forever!

Did I mention that I decided to never diet again? That has been the key to my success. Diets are no more than anvils hanging over our heads waiting to crash. We eat food that we do not like and drink excessive amounts of water in an effort to take the weight off immediately. When I followed the "diet of the month's" directive to drink at least eight glasses of water per day, I felt like I had to pee all of the time. Sorry, that is not a feeling that I desire or enjoy. It's diet nonsense that will end in a crash.

One day I had Oprah on and her guest was Doctor Oz, who seemed like a genuinely friendly guy who made a lot of sense. But then he handed Oprah some drink concoction that he and his kids drink for breakfast. Oprah tasted it and made the same face that Lucy Ricardo made in the famous Vitameatavegamin episode. The man made a lot of good points, but I'm passing on that stuff and having oatmeal and fresh fruit instead. I enjoy those. What we need to do is take a look at how a truly normal person eats and drinks. They do not exist by doing the kooky things that we do when we diet. Losing weight is a simple numbers game. Eat above our daily calorie needs we gain weight, eat below and we lose. There is absolutely no magic here, and most likely never will be. If we are waiting for the magic pill, we are going to be fat for a long time. The good news is that we can eat what we like, as long as it is below the threshold. I go back to my first diet with the pork chop fried in

Crisco: I lost lots of weight. Now I am not suggesting that approach, but it will work. Good balanced nutrition is what is best.

EXERCISE

I glossed over how much I disliked gym class when I spoke about school and sports earlier. "Hate" summed it up. I hated the exercise and that fact that we were forced to parade as a naked pack into the showers after each class. Not showering was not an option. I despised gym so much that I failed it in tenth grade by showing up without a uniform or being caught not showering. That meant I had to take it four times per week in eleventh grade. I resorted to lying to the school nurse about back pain. I used that excuse a few times and was told that I would need a doctor's excuse in the future. I was out of free rides. So I went to my family doctor and went through the same routine about my back. I was able to get out of gym for the year; ditto my senior year.

The contribution of exercise in weight loss is often overblown. Have you ever truly calculated how many calories you burn with a twenty minute walk? My pedometer says 145 calories. An average peanut butter Easter egg is 300 calories! Unless you are committed to a few hours of exercise per day, your weight loss directly depends on your caloric intake.

Many people use exercise to continue to take in too many calories. In fact, I did no exercise while losing my first 100 pounds and bragged about it! Then the vision of my mother and great grandfather in wheelchairs at the end of their lives made me realize that I was wrong. I have been blessed with a family lineage that boasts obese people with no cholesterol, blood pressure, or diabetes issues, living well into their late eighties and early nineties. But the last five years of life were either tough getting around or wheelchair bound. I knew that exercise would be my best shot at avoiding that fate.

I joined a gym. The owners were wonderful and I learned a few things, but it was not for me. I just hated going there after working all day. I started to work out lifting dumbbells and doing deep-knee bends during the newscasts on my radio show. I was doing the talking the rest of the time, but had nearly ten minutes at the top of the hour and six at the bottom. My co-workers poked a little fun on the air, but within a few months my muscles were nicely developed, and I could easily pick up fifty pound bags of salt. I cut my own lawn, which is a three mile walk at a brisk pace.

This year I made two resolutions: to exercise and cook more. Now I walk a minimum of two miles per day along with my dumbbell regimen. Do I feel better? You bet I do! And once I got used to being active, it drove me crazy to sit on my can. When we sit, we want to eat. When we are doing other things, we do not have time. Pretty basic, but very true.

BINGES AND DEMONS

Never dieting again means acknowledging that there are times that we are can take a break and let our hair down. I had pre-meditated dinners where I was going to eat something that was heavier in calories, including dessert, than I would normally consume. This made it seem less like a diet and more like I had changed the way I eat. Normal weight people eat these things, just not continually and every day. We can go to a wedding reception and have all of the goodies and the cake, but just one normal serving.

We Americans love our huge portions. That is why we have huge bottoms. The tough part is keeping this eating to once in a while. In the past, this always lead to once per week, then twice, then failure and back to our old ways. That is the risk we take if we do not have the proper mindset.

The best laid plans go awry when the food demons come for us. They haunt every single day. Just like the Emperor called Luke to the dark side in Star Wars, the food demons remind me how enjoyable three candy bars and three packs of snack cakes at one setting would be. The food demons will try to take over the steering of our vehicles, taking them through a more convenient than ever drive-thru of some sort. This is where I needed prayer to focus on the fact that I was already eating what I liked and did not need all of this extra nonsense, that family and my goals were much more important, and that food ruled me for fifty years, and it would no longer! I am stronger than food. Overeaters Anonymous calls it "my higher power", for me that is Christ. I rely on prayer to get me through. There have been times when the demons were driving and I gave them the boot and took back the steering wheel. That feeling is much better than the taste of any junk food. If we do not give up the romance for food, we will always be fat.

EATING AT THE DROP OF A HAT

Being powerless over food is the root of every compulsive overeater's issues. Food is what rules everything, yet we deny its power. We come up with every excuse imaginable to reason away why we overeat. Some say, "I eat when I'm depressed, I eat to celebrate, I eat when I am stressed, blah, blah, blah." Well, I am a compulsive overeater, and I eat at the drop of a hat, and so do you! We make these excuses without ever really doing self-inventory.

Take a serious look at what we consume daily, weekly, monthly—most overeaters will see just how obscene it is. Food drove me for years. I had to know what the next meal would be while I was eating this one. Around four pm I'd ask my wife what we were having for dinner, she would often reply with an, "I don't know." How could she not know? This is dinner we're talking about here! Bonnie likes food, but it does not drive her. She can eat half of a candy bar and save the other half for another time. I want all of it now, and two more. She doesn't plan it that way. It is the way she eats naturally, and it's the reason that she can fit into her wedding dress.

We have to get over food. Our brains are the greatest computers ever developed and yet food controls us. Too bad there isn't anti-virus software for the brain that would repair this addiction. We reason our addiction away the same way that people addicted to drugs and alcohol do. It's one of the reasons that the diet meetings did not work for me. People sit around in misery relating how deprived they are.

According to Dictionary.com, there are two basic definitions for addiction: the first is, "to become physiologically or psychologically dependent on a habit forming substance." The second is, "to occupy oneself with or involve oneself in something habitually or compulsively." Compulsive overeaters fit both definitions a-to-z. "But it's hard, we have to eat." Yes, we do, but we do not have to overeat! Take back your life! The Eagles song "Already Gone" has a great line that pertains directly to compulsive overeaters: "So often times it happens that we live our lives in chains and we never even know we have the key."

Every excuse in the book has been used to explain overeating. At some point they are all just excuses, either we take a stand or continue to grow in size. It amazes me how many preachers speak to drug and alcohol issues, while ignoring gluttony, which is mentioned many times throughout the Bible. Some of the most prominent preachers on TV today are morbidly obese. Unless they changed the Bible recently, that is a true sin. We are the gate keepers. In order to change, we first have to admit that we are powerless over food. Will our food addictions lead to heart issues, diabetes, knee and joint replacement, or a scooter chair? If we do not give up the addictive romance that we have for food, we will be fat forever.

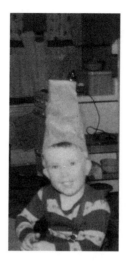 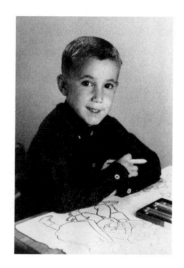

R.J. Harris at age 4   R.J. Harris in second grade

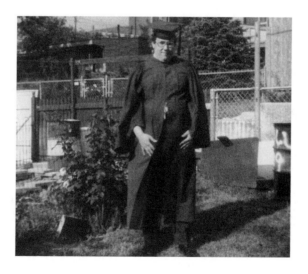

R.J. Harris: graduation in June 1972

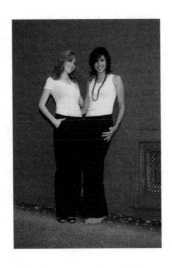

Models in R.J.'s size 58 jeans

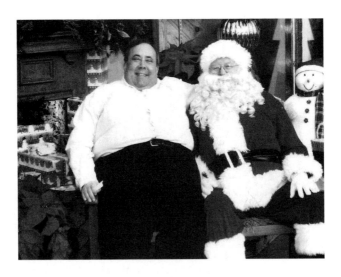

R.J. Harris with Santa in 2005

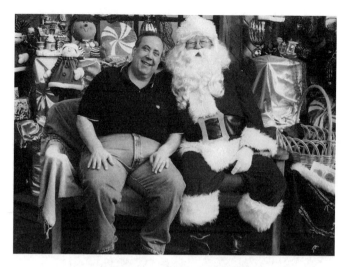

R.J. Harris with Santa in 2006

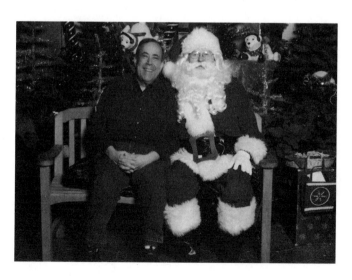

R.J. Harris with Santa in 2007

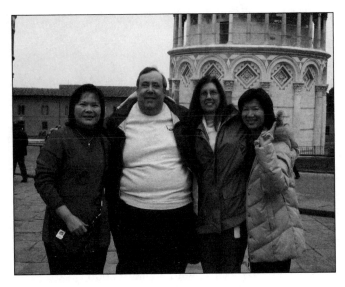

R.J., Bonnie and the women from Taiwan in Pisa, Italy

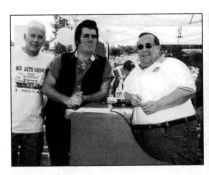

R.J. Harris with Elvis tribute
artist Ronnie Allyn in August
1999

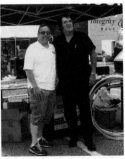

R.J. Harris with Elvis
tribute artist Ronnie
Allyn in August 2009

WEIGHT LOSS TERRORISTS

Losing weight is never easy. Most times the same people who believe that we should lose weight are the first to try and derail us, another reason to never diet again. Change your eating habits and tell nobody. When you announce a diet, the saboteurs come out immediately to entice you to eat a little extra on this special occasion or outing. Say nothing and nobody will notice. Simple, but it works.

My mother, who was obese, would say, "Richie, you need to reduce," with her Pennsylvania Dutch accent, then the next minute try to feed me. There are others who want you to fail so that they are not alone, for they, too, are compulsive overeaters. For once in your dieting life, let actions speak louder than words. People will eventually catch on that you are losing weight and will ask if you are dieting. I would say no, that I am just watching what I eat and eating smaller portions. To most this does not seem like dieting and they relent.

Be aware that folks try to derail you all along the way. I wish I had a five-dollar-bill for every person who told me that I don't have any more weight to lose, when I still had fifty pounds to go. I would say, "So you think that I should just be fifty-pounds overweight, is that right?" Fifty pounds over is obese. Stick to your goal; don't let complements lull you into remaining overweight.

Keep in mind that I have been saying all along that you need to eat what you enjoy. So at Thanksgiving and other family holidays, I ate traditional turkey and potatoes, but also a tablespoon of the vegetable casseroles, and other calorie-laden foods. I know that it is hard to believe, but that's all I needed. I have a rather thin friend who says he eats until he is no longer hungry, rather than until he is full. He credits that approach to being rather thin all of his life. People who are naturally trim share some important traits: food does not drive them, and they consume portions that are on the smaller size. These portions are normal, but most Americans cannot fathom that in the age of the sixty-four ounce convenience store soda tankard. We want extra large everything and think that it is normal. For years my wife would suggest sharing a dessert. Are you kidding me? I want every morsel of mine; get your own! Now I am enjoying sharing dessert with her. I enjoy eating like she does now.

IT AIN'T EASY BEING FAT,
BUT THAT'S YOUR PROBLEM

Nothing amuses me more than "The National Association to Advance Fat Acceptance" (NAAFA.) Obese people will never be accepted. Get over it. You are what you are; either accept that you are fat and the judgment that comes with it, or lose weight. It is human nature to judge others. We do it naturally in so many areas. I have heard fat people judge other fat people. If you are not the fattest person in the room, the fattest is the target. Some people even refuse to think they are fat. They put on ten pounds per year and five years later they are obese, but they continue to judge fat people. No politically correct organization is going to change human nature.

One day at the checkout at a local drug store

every parent's worst nightmare happened. A cute girl of four or five years of age said, "Mommy, this man is really fat!" I knew that the mother was ready to run and hide, until I said, "You are correct. I became so fat because I eat way too much. That is why you need to listen to your mother when she tells you that you had enough to eat or no more candy. If you listen and eat properly, you will not become fat like me." I could see the relief on the mother's face. Hey, I was fat because of me. Out of the mouths of babes comes the truth!

We do face humiliation when we are obese: having to ask for a seat belt extension on the plane, never being able to fit thru a turnstile, staying off rides at amusement parks because the safety bar will crush our fat stomachs, or never being able to fit in a desk at our child's open house at school. Even some of the "one on one" weight loss programs that I attended were humiliating. I remember being too big for the scale at one of these programs.

They herded me back to a rustic looking freight scale that the owner must have picked up at an auction. It was the kind that they had at train stations when I was a kid. Imagine the embarrassment of being too fat for the regular scale at a weight loss clinic!

In March 2006 I escorted forty-six of my listeners on a trip to Rome and the Tuscany region of Italy; I decided that my life would change the day that I stepped off the plane upon our return. While in Italy I already started to slow up. I did not go wild or binge. I did enjoy the wine! While at the Leaning Tower in Pisa, two Taiwanese women, who did not speak a lick of English, came up to me, amazed at how big I was. I could tell by their mannerisms that I was the fattest person they had ever seen close up. One rubbed my belly like I was Buddha and wanted to have her photo taken with me. I obliged with a big smile. While I would have been happy to anyway, it was extra sweet knowing that this would be among my last photos of being nearly 400 pounds. I had one taken for me as well. By the way, I only made it a few floors up into the tower before I was out of breath and could no longer hack it. Bonnie made it all the way. Some day I will return and see the view from the top!

I have always known that my weight issue was just that: mine! Addicts who continue to blame other people and things will always be addicts. That means that you will always be fat. If being fat is your choice, be all right with it and all that comes with it. Any anger should not be directed at others, but rather the root of the problem: you.

FAT PEOPLE ARE LAZY!

Sorry, it's true. Fat people become experts at making one trip. I was an accomplished juggler considering how many different items I could carry just so that I would not have to make two trips, whether the load had to travel twenty feet or twenty blocks. Many times I juggled so many items that I would drop things and start muttering and cursing. But did I change my ways? No, that would mean more effort. This skill did come in handy once, as I am the all-time champion of the pumpkin carry event at a local garden center. The competition was to see who could carry the most pumpkins at once. Using my girth and lazy man carrying skills, I set a record of twenty-seven pumpkins, which still stands today.

It was standard operating procedure to

avoid all steps. Heaven forbid I would have to go up or down one flight of steps at home to get something. I would grow angry when realizing that I had forgotten something resulting in having to make two trips. At work I took the elevator in a building that had only two floors.

Yes, I had a great work ethic all along, and I would go rock hunting and such, but I was truly lazy at heart, sitting around and watching many hours of TV. Like most fat folks, I would circle parking lots to get the closest spots, like a buzzard circling a carcass. Now I park as far away as I can.

YOU ALWAYS HURT THE ONES YOU LOVE

Step eight in the Alcoholics Anonymous twelve step program calls for the need to make a list of people you had harmed and become willing to make amends to them all. It is easy to see how an alcoholic could rack up a rather lengthy list, but who do we fat people hurt, other than ourselves? Our families!

As a kid I was always at the pool; I was a water bug. As a dad, I never went to the pool, except when we had our own in California. I was never able to participate in sports, because I was lousy at best. When we went to eat we had to wait for a table, because I could not fit in a booth. I remember the family being loaded on the back of a ride at Universal Studios like cattle because I could not fit in a regular seat on the ride. We were put in the handicapped section because I was handicapped by mass.

Don't get me wrong, I was a cub master for my two boys, a soccer referee, confirmation and Sunday school teacher, but physical things were out. My three children all played sports and except for that short stint as a soccer referee, I could only support them through being an active spectator at their sporting events. My daughter Christi recently shared her fear that I would have to escort her down the aisle in a scooter at her wedding.

The other way that it took its toll was that I was the head shark when it came to food. I guarded every extra piece of food in sight, just short of shouting, "It's mine, all mine" like a pirate does with his treasure. Bonnie and I had many spirited discussions over my obsession with food. It may not be as devastating as drugs and alcohol at first glance, but tell that to your loved ones when you die at a young age from heart failure.

THE SYMBOLS OF VICTORY

My overall goal was to weigh 195 pounds. But I set smaller goals each step along the way. I had two categories: pounds and waist size. I weighed myself every morning without fail. My goal centered on twenty-five pound increments. Weight Watchers awarded a magnet for each of those steps. My twenty-five, fifty, seventy-five and one-hundred pound magnets still adorn my refrigerator, along with three photos of me and Santa Claus. In the first photo I hardly fit on the bench with Santa, the second and third show amazing progress. It's rather ironic that over the years I was called on to play Santa often, but Santa suits were too small for me. Yes, I was so big there was no Santa suit in my size. Once when I played against the Harlem Globetrotters as a Washington

General, a special suit had to be made for me by the promotion director of the radio station. There was nothing even close that would fit.

Now I never have to worry about that again. I proudly throw the big & tall catalogs in the trash. When I got to a forty-two inch waist I knew that I would never go to the "fat boy" store again. That was a huge victory. Big & tall catalogs still arrive in the mail, only to hit the trash can with the flick of a wrist. It takes some getting used to. I look at the opening in my pants and still think that I won't fit, but I do with room to spare. Being able to eat on an airplane and buckle my seat belt without an extension are also big victories. Before, I never had to return my tray table to an upright position, I was too fat to ever use it. And how embarrassing is it to have to ask a flight attendant for a seat belt extension every time? I also, at my biggest had to order extensions for my vehicle belts. Nothing was simple. That is now history; this victory tastes sweeter than any food on Earth.

EVERY DIET WORKS

My standard line is that every diet works. It's true; people can lose weight on the cabbage soup diet, ice cream diet, banana diet, and all of the other off-beat tricks that humans think will be the magic answer to weight loss. On any given week at the checkout line there are several of these miracle diets headlined on the magazine rack. Usually they are the "secret" diets of the stars, all of whom have to lose a whopping five to ten pounds. Remember, losing weight is a pure numbers game. An average banana is eighty calories. Assuming that your target is to consume 1,500 calories, you can have almost nineteen bananas per day and lose weight. How long do you really think this will work for you? How much cabbage soup will you consume before you go crazy?

These mono-diets are pure nonsense. If you have a sizeable amount of weight to lose, you do not stand a chance of succeeding. I've known folks who thought that they would just kick-start their loss with one of these kooky diets, only to have it all sputter out quickly.

I loved the Atkins diet; what man wouldn't? I had bacon every day for months. You would figure that a carnivore would never tire of it. I got to the point where I could not look at another piece of bacon, or cheese for that matter. Everything is about balance and variety. Then there are the medical diet aids. One has spotty uncontrollable bowel movements, which may cause underwear staining as a side effect. Let me see, eating a good balanced diet or doing a number two without warning in my pants? I think I'll go for a good eating plan. How about you?

You have to decide if your diet is for managing weight or changing the way you eat forever.

Weight management is trying to control the yo-yo with on again, off again diets. Changing forever means weight loss that will stick. People continue to pay billions of dollars each year for gimmicks that will allow them to remain in the yo-yo cycle forever, when a balanced program of foods that you like is all that you need and costs nothing. If you are waiting for the silver-bullet to end obesity, you will be fat forever.

GETTING RID OF THE SCARS

One morning I played a commercial for Stratis-Gayner Plastic Surgery on my radio show, a new practice run by two experienced area plastic surgeons. Doctor Stratis focused on the body, while Doctor Gayner focused on the face. Their campaign motivated me to call them. No matter what type of exercise you commit to, once you have weighed several hundred pounds for a length of time, you have skin that will never tighten, inches of it. I decided that I simply did not want to look at those scars every day. Any scars plastic surgery would leave behind would be more palatable than looking at inches of flab still hanging around after accomplishing that much weight loss.

My meeting with the doctors was everything that I had hoped for, and we decided on a two-prong approach. The first surgery would be "gyno-plasty" (male breast reduction), "smart lipo" and some tightening of the neck. Six months later we tackled "abdomoplasty" (tummy tuck) and a maxxlift (neck lift) to get rid of my turkey neck. And finally a posterior body lift one year later. For me the procedures were a breeze, and I would do it again in one second! Along with the weight loss, this made me feel like a new man! As with any medical procedure, choosing the right doctors is the key. I also benefited from my dumbbell work-outs, as my chest and abdomen were pretty muscu-lar before I had the procedures. Doctor Stratis never touched my muscles, making recovery time next to nothing. In each case I did it over a long holiday weekend and went back to work on time.

I truly believe that looking at the rolls of flab every day would have eventually sent me into a psychological tailspin. While this may not be for everyone, it allowed me to move to a whole new level mentally. I now endorse Stratis-Gayner Plastic Surgery with commercials on my radio show and have received quite a bit of feedback from fellow former fatties that who rid themselves of their weight loss scars.

KEY POINTS

Eat three normal meals

Yes that means a good breakfast. It does start there, just like you've been told all of these years. Want to continue to use every excuse under the sun as to why you cannot eat breakfast? Go ahead... and continue to be fat. Never eat in front of the TV or in the car. Take time to enjoy your meals.

Embrace and eat fruits and vegetables

Fruits are as sweet and refreshing as any candy you find. I mean it! Why do you think candy often mimics fruit flavors? Because fruit is fantastic! Even in winter there are many fresh delicacies to be had. I usually do one fresh pineapple per week during the cold months. Sweet and fantastic!

Vegetables get a bad rap. Prepared and seasoned properly they are wonderful. Squash, zucchini, egg-plant, green beans, peas, carrots, sweet potato, or any other potato that you love. Lots of sweet corn in summer! Just don't overdo the starches, and account for everything. I eat about two potatoes per week. I limit corn also. Often I put the veggies on the grill with the meat I'm cooking. Just awesome!

Weigh and measure everything

Do just what it says. We love to lie to ourselves. Just an extra this or that. It adds up quickly. Then we say, "I don't understand why I'm not losing weight. I'm eating what I should be." An extra this and that becomes a lot of extra this and that by the end of a day, a week, a month. You have to be hon-est and weigh it all! I did it religiously for the first 100 pounds and still weigh meat today. You will be surprised how much you get when you eat a cup of fresh blueberries or strawberries.

Write down all that you eat

Once again this is about honesty and accountability. Accountability for YOU. Lying to yourself is the issue here. You cannot lie to others. Time will show your lies through your continued weight gain. It does not take long for others to see the lies. Log what you eat and its cost. There are a million great calorie counter books in stores and free calorie counters online. In a recent 13-week study, folks who kept a record of what they ate lost 3.5 pounds more than those who did not. Write it down—every morsel.

Weigh yourself daily

The scale is not your enemy; it is your conscience.

When you weigh yourself every day, it will not take a week or month to see that you are out of whack. Staying off the scale is another way that we lie to ourselves. Out of sight, out of mind, until D-Day approaches and for whatever reason you have to get on a scale. There will be days when that scale goes up a bit. That is natural.

Eat what you love

Look, if you are going to change for life, you have to like what you eat. I eat real butter, use half & half in my coffee, and real mayonnaise. Most quick-loss diets require you to limit things like bananas. Bananas are my favorite fruit and I eat one every day. Come on, it's fruit for Pete's sake. You are going to have to navigate the rest of your life eating sensibly; you'll end up like the Titanic if you force yourself to eat foods that do not satisfy.

Biggie size nothing

Our biggest issue in America is portion size. You do not need a biggie anything or combo meal. I have talked myself into combo meals because the price difference was pennies. Why pass up the deal? The price difference was pennies; the caloric cost was in the hundreds. Five ounces of steak and half of a huge baking potato is enough to fill. Really, it is. You must be strong at restaurants. Researchers found that people ate eighty-five percent more bread when their server offered them seconds. Just say no to any extras!

Be honest

That is what the last few steps are all about. Be honest with yourself. You can hide your eating from others, but they will see through you as your waistline grows. This has to be about you. Are you willing to take the steps required to be honest about every detail of what you eat?

Find a Hobby/Don't Sit Around/Get Outside

Studies have shown that Americans are most likely to go off a diet between seven and midnight. If your current hobby is sitting in front of the TV, you will probably continue to binge eat. Like smoking is associated with drinking by many, food and TV are the same. Find something that interests you and get busy. Even if you choose a rather sedentary hobby, you will be keeping busy and away from food.

Every Day/Hour Counts

If you slip, get back to eating properly immediately. Do not wait until tomorrow. Never again wait for Monday to begin eating correctly. Every minute of every day counts. Every minute that you wait is another in the pit of addiction!

Pray/Talk Yourself Out of It

Weekly and sometimes daily I pray to the Lord to help me pass by drive-thru windows and convenience stores. I will have made up my mind to stop, just this once. Prayer and a good common sense talking-to-myself session have kept me on the right path so many times. At times I say out loud, "Just go home, go home!" And I do.

Never Diet Again

Change your lifestyle. It is the only way to succeed and be happy. A recent survey published in *Women's Health* showed that 30.9% of women surveyed admitted to being on three to six diets in the past two years. Change your lifestyle and break the yo-yo diet cycle for good. If you eat healthier with smaller portions, you will lose weight. You really do not need the junk and all of its calories and will learn to be satisfied by a normal amount of food in short fashion. Eat until you are no longer hungry, not until you are full.

Also remember that this is not a race. You put the weight on slowly, do not expect to take it off quickly. We put on five-pounds over a period of months or years, then expect it to be gone in one week. I averaged weight loss of two-pounds per week, excellent results while eating what I love.

Cook

A recent study showed that young adults who frequently made their own meals had much healthier diets than their peers who had never set foot in the kitchen. These same folks bought more fresh vegetables each week as well. Embrace the food that you eat. Pour some of the passion for food into the challenge of making new, wonderful tasting foods that excite you and the family. Trust me when I tell you that your wife will not mind. I do lots of cooking on the grill. I have made many vegetable delicacies outside on the grill. It is a blast!

Get Help

I called the ladies from Weight Watchers my "parole officers." I could not have made it without them. While meetings were not my cup of tea, their encouragement and the Weight Watchers program were essential for me. Overeaters Anonymous is also a wonderful program that works for many.

TOP REASONS TO LOSE

Better love life

Study after study shows it. Don't need to elaborate.

No more BIG & Tall or PLUS Size stores

Wear the latest styles. Dress the way you've always wanted to.

For your health

Your risk of everything bad increases when you are fat. Is a scooter chair at a young age in your future?

Save money

On gas, clothing, food, and health care.

Example for your children

Kids with fat parents are fat as well. Again, study after study shows it.

Indigestion is gone

No more sleepless nights with acid reflux.

No more snoring

Who needs a CPAP machine?

For YOU!

It has to be for YOU! If you want to do it for any-one else, or any other reason, you will fail! This is about YOU!

IT FEELS GREAT TO BE FIT

My fellow radio host Rush Limbaugh spoke frequently about exercise having no impact on weight loss that it is all about what you eat. Earlier you read that I believe the same. But at some point you learn that exercise, no matter how much, makes you feel better. It is just the plain truth. Even Rush has changed his tune on exercise and spends time daily on a treadmill.

The following is an easy to stick with dumbbell workout created by my friend Mark Noble. Mark is a listener and supporter of mine. He has cheered me on every step of the way and inspired me with this program. Remember, you do not need to do all of it at one time. Pick different parts to do on different days. Only do as many reps as you can to start. Build up over time. Keep a journal every day with how many reps you did and at what weight, so you'll be able to see your improvement. I'm sure there are things you won't be able to do. Just do what you can and what feels comfortable. Make sure to use the treadmill or take a walk or jog daily. A little more and a little faster every week.

*<u>Six Point Dumbbell Press</u>: (2 sets of 10 reps if possible or whatever is comfortable). Hold dumbbells at your side. Curl them up to your shoulders. Turn dumb bells to face forward. Press straight up over your head. Bring back down to shoulders. Turn dumb bells so ends are facing out. Curl back down to sides.

*<u>Swing Backs</u>: (2 sets of 10 reps if possible or whatever is comfortable). Hold dumbbells at your side. Keep arms straight and extend them backwards as far as possible. Return dumbbells to your

side (make sure to make a complete stop before doing the next rep).

*Straight Lifts: (2 sets of 10 reps). Hold dumbbells at your side. Simply pull dumbbells straight up to armpits, and then back down.

*Chop Wood: (1 set of 10 each side). Hold dumbbell with both hands up by neck resting on shoulder. Twist and bend in wood chopping motion first to the right 10 times then to the left 10 times.

*Front Rises: (2 sets of 10 each side alternating). Hold weights in front of you resting them on thighs. Alternate lifting dumbbells, right then left and over again 10 times, straight up and out, keeping arms straight.

*Tees: (2 sets of 10). Hold dumbbells at sides. Lift to form T and back to sides.

*<u>Push-ups</u>: (if possible). Do the kind where you get on your knees and just do a couple of sets of push-ups. Increase reps, as you get stronger.

*<u>Military Twists</u>: (1 set of 10). Hold weights at shoulders. Alternate lifting dumbbells right to left while twisting torso. (Twist to side that you are lifting dumb bell with).

*<u>Dips</u>: Stand between two chairs. Place hands on tops of chairs. Dip body down then back up.

*<u>Curls</u>: 4 sets of 10

*<u>Behind the Head:</u> 20 reps behind the head.

*<u>Rows</u>: (1 set of 20 each side). Put knee on bench. Place hand on bench. With other hand pull weight from floor up to chest. Switch sides do other arm.

*Obliques: (1set of 10). Hold dumbbells at each side. Alternate bending side-to-side.

*Squats: (2 sets of 10). Hold weights at side. Bend knees and then stand straight back up.

*Straight Leg Dead Lifts: (2 sets of 10). Hold weights in front of you. Keep legs straight, bend forward (like doing a toe touch) and then stand straight back up.

This workout has helped me build a positive attitude. It feels great to be fit. I also recommend *Tiki Barber's Pure Hard Workout: Stop Wasting Time and Start Building Real Strength and Muscle* by Tiki Barber and Joe Carini. While this book is very hardcore, it contains many great exercises that will complement Mark Noble's dumbbell routine. It throws some exciting twists into your routine.

There is no need to invest any significant amount of money into workout equipment; you can find anything that you need at local yard sales for pennies on the dollar. The first commitment I made in this process was to never diet again, the second was to never buy new exercise equipment again. Been there, done that. It is all available for next to nothing. Be patient and look around.

Add a one-mile walk five days per week and you will feel great. The entire routine will take you thirty to forty minutes per day without having to join anything or go anywhere.

For years I acted as master of ceremonies for many charity walk-a-thons but never walked in one. Now I walk in many events and raise money. It has been a true pleasure to be a spokesperson for the American Heart and Stroke Associations "Start" walking program.

IT IS TIME. YOU CAN DO IT!

Most of you read this book because you are obese, or at the very least overweight. If you identified with any of my journey there is a good chance that you are addicted to food. Special diets to lose weight date back centuries. William the Conqueror allegedly pioneered the single food or drink diet. In the early 1900s they sold tapeworms as weight loss aids. Millions have gone bonkers trying to lose weight since Dr. Lulu Hunt Peters introduced the word "calorie" to the world in 1918. There is no silver bullet. Not now, nor in the foreseeable future. We food addicts hope, pray, and fantasize about a pill that will allow us to gorge. If you continue to wait, you will die fat.

One glance around most any public setting in

the United States will show you how serious this issue is. The majority of us will be on our way to obesity if we continue at this rate. I'm simply pointing out that this is real, and you and I are not alone. But will you admit that you are addicted? That you are powerless over your addiction to eating and that it controls you? Will you allow food to overrule the most powerful part of our bodies—the brain? Will you check your ego at the door and enter a world of new possibilities?

Abstinence is sweet! It is like paying bills on time and never worrying about bill collectors calling. It's just one of those things that makes life better. I understand why people get such a rush over scaling a mountain. This is the same rush, a true sense of accomplishment and control. The day that you truly make up your mind to change forever will be a monumental one. You will feel better immediately!

This is about YOU! Decide that you are going

to be the very best person that you can for YOU. This is not a show for others; they will see the results, or lack of, very plainly. You must stop lying to yourself! How many diets have you been on? How much weight have you lost and gained? Why will your next diet work when none have to date? You have not succeeded, and you will not succeed until you change forever.

The good news is that eating properly forever does not mean that you eat rabbit food all of your life. Eat what you love. Just account for what you eat every day of your life. In this case you can have your cake (weight loss) and eat it too.

In the Disney/Pixar Academy-Award-winning mega-hit *WALL-E*, humans who live in space on a "starliner" become totally reliant on machinery and suffer severe bone loss from years of consuming food, becoming severely obese and being unable to walk, and are now living on floating recliners. Look around you my friends. Every year more

Americans achieve obesity. Every year we have more limpers, walkers, and scooters, among those who would not have the need if they were normal weight. The writers of *WALL-E* were obviously inspired by what they see in America today. There is not one week that goes by without seeing a butts-and-guts obesity story on network TV news. You know the stories about how fat we are and how obesity is killing us, where they only show mid-body shots of big buts and huge guts—no faces.

You can make a choice right now. Yes, NOW! Take control over food. Begin eating properly for the rest of your life today. You have it within you to become a success story. You can be one of those who truly beats the odds. You can be someone who is admired for what you have accomplished. You will feel great! This will be your Mt. Everest!

Never diet again. There are over 28,000 ways to lose weight, but only one works. You know what it is. Now do it!

You will always be fat if you say:

- No matter how hard I try, I just cannot eat breakfast.
- If only I had time to exercise, I wouldn't gain weight.
- But I love to eat.
- I'm on the road and cannot eat healthy.
- I cannot give up my beer.
- It's so hard.
- It's my birthday.
- It's the drugs that I take.
- I feel left out.
- I will start my diet on Monday.

Suggested Reading

- *Mindless Eating* by Brian Wansink, PH.D.
- *Tiki Barber's Pure Hard Workout: Stop Wasting Time and Start Building Real Strength and Muscle* by Tiki Barber and Joe Carini
- *Alcoholics Anonymous Big Book*
- *The Biggest Loser Complete Calorie Counter* by Cheryl Forberg, RD
- *The Skinny On: Willpower* by Jim Randel
- *Life Is Tremendous* by Charles "Tremendous" Jones